HEALTH
and
BEAUTY

HEALTH
and
BEAUTY

MARY ROSE QUIGG

CHARTWELL
BOOKS. INC

Published by
CHARTWELL BOOKS, INC.
A Division of BOOK SALES, INC.
P.O. Box 7100
114 Northfield Avenue
Edison, New Jersey 08818-7100

Text © Mary Rose Quigg 1995
Layout and Design © Sunburst Books 1995

ISBN 0-7858-0445-5

Printed and bound in China

PUBLISHER'S NOTE
The publisher does not take any responsibility for
the implementation of any recommendations, ideas and
techniques in this book. They should not be regarded as
substitutes for the advice of a qualified medical practitioner
or other qualified professional. Any use to which the
recommendations, ideas and techniques are put is at the
reader's sole discretion and risk.

CONTENTS

INTRODUCTION

In a world of increasingly 'green' concerns, many people are shunning the extravagant claims of the high-tech health and beauty industries and welcoming a return to the pure, natural world of kitchen cosmetics. If, like them, you are looking for simple, inexpensive remedies to create in your own home, then this is the book for you.

The *Health and Beauty* handguide contains a wealth of traditional hints and tips on care of the face and body, stress reduction, essential first-aid, and healthy eating. Many of the preparations have been passed down through the generations to me; others are the result of my own experience and my experiments with the treasure trove of natural ingredients that are so easily available to us today.

Alongside a collection of luxurious recipes with which to pamper yourself in moments of relaxation, you will find a directory to some of the mystifying terminology adopted by the food and cosmetic industries.

In today's hectic world, *Health and Beauty* provides invaluable suggestions for creating a healthy environment in your home and improving the quality of your daily beauty care without recourse to mass-produced synthetic products.

CARE OF THE BODY FROM HEAD TO TOE

Hair Care

Good hair care starts at home in the way you treat your hair. Always brush the hair before washing to remove tangles and any surface dirt.

To avoid splitting hair, start combing the ends first and work your way upwards. Do not start at the roots. Use bristle brushes in preference to nylon as they reduce static and distribute the oils more evenly. Avoid brushing or combing your hair too often as this can cause the hair to split.

Choose the proper shampoo. Frequent-wash brands can be used daily on oily or normal hair. A rich creamy shampoo is best for hair that has been chemically treated with a perm or colour. If you suffer from dandruff then use special treatment shampoos but only while the problem persists, as they dry out the hair. There are many homemade shampoos for every hair type. You will find some of these in this book.

To wash hair: use warm water to wet the hair, put a small blob of shampoo on the palms of the hands and smooth it gently over the hair. Lather the shampoo with the pads of your fingers. Use this massaging action on the scalp for about a minute. If your hair is long, only lather the scalp. The rest will be washed as you rinse.

Unless the hair is very dirty, one shampoo wash is sufficient. A lot of lather means the product is high in detergent - it doesn't reflect the quality. Avoid tangles by letting the hair fall naturally. Wet hair is weaker and more easily damaged than dry, so treat gently. Always rinse thoroughly – the water should run clear and the hair feel 'squeaky'.

All hair types appreciate a conditioning rinse; normal and fine hair will benefit from a weekly treatment, while dry and chemically-treated hair will need an application after every shampoo. After washing hair, towel dry and then gently comb your conditioner through the hair. Leave for a few minutes before rinsing thoroughly.

As with a shampoo, choose a conditioner to suit your type of hair. Intensive conditioning treatments should be given at least once a month. These are richer than ordinary conditioners and are left on the hair instead of being rinsed out.

Hair can stretch up to a third of its length when wet but return to normal when dry. If hair is wrapped tightly around rollers or circular brushes during blow-drying, it can make the hair brittle. Do not constantly keep hair tied back tightly as this can lead to thinning around the hairline.

Overuse of hair dryers can parch the hair, so don't use the hottest setting and stop when the hair is still slightly damp. Where possible let the hair dry naturally, but not in the sun, as the wet hair absorbs the ultra violet rays which can damage the hair. Avoid using heated rollers, curling tongs or the hair dryer every day, and also over-treating with chemicals such as bleach and perm lotions.

Consult a reputable hair salon for the best products to use on problem hair. Hair should be trimmed every six weeks – each strand is like a piece of rope and when it splits it is like a rope unravelling. Cutting the hair is the only way to seal the ends.

Natural Hair Care

For an effective cleansing rinse: squeeze the juice of a lemon into 300 ml/½ pint brown ale and apply to damp hair. Massage well and leave for a few minutes then rinse thoroughly.

To combat scurf: add 10 ml/2 tsp cider vinegar to two beaten egg yolks. Pour 150 ml/¼ pint boiling water over 60 ml/4 tbsp dried rosemary and infuse for an hour. Strain and add 30 ml/2 tbsp each olive oil and castor oil. Massage into wet hair and leave for 10 minutes. Rinse well. Alternatively, soak 60 ml/1 pint nettle leaves in 600 ml/1 pint boiling water for four hours. Strain, add 125 ml/¼ pint cider vinegar. Massage daily into the scalp.

As a hair rinse: pour 600 ml/1 pint boiling water over 30 ml/2 tbsp fresh rosemary leaves or 5 ml/1 tbsp dried rosemary, leave for 15 minutes and strain. After rinsing off the shampoo pour the preparation over the hair and towel dry.

Alternatively, use 30 ml/2 tbsp cider vinegar and 15 ml/1 tbsp rose water added to 1.2 litre/2 pints warm water.

For a hair tonic: soak 50 g/2 oz nettles, 25 g/1 oz rosemary and 25 g/1 oz marigold petals in 250 ml/ 8 fl oz vodka for three weeks. Strain and add three drops lavender oil and 100 ml/4 fl oz distilled water. Massage this into the hair and scalp three times every week.

To highlight brown hair: bring out the natural highlights in dark hair by rinsing it with beer or red wine.

Boil 30 ml/2 tbsp dried rosemary and 30 ml/2 tbsp dried sage in 1.2 litre/2 pints water. Cover and simmer for 10 minutes. Leave for two hours, strain and add 150 ml/¼ pint cider vinegar. Bottle the mixture and pour on wet, clean hair frequently.

To highlight blonde hair: use the above method but substitute 60 ml/4 tbsp camomile for the herbs.

To add body to fine dry hair: beat one or two egg yolks with 5 ml/1 tsp mild shampoo. Wet hair with tepid water and shampoo hair with mixture. Rinse well with lukewarm water.

Caring For Your Ears

Small glands in the outer ear canal are constantly producing wax to protect the sensitive lining of the ear from infection. The soft wax is continually being brushed out by tiny hairs. Sometimes it can harden and block the outer ear, causing deafness.

Do not attempt to remove wax with cotton wool buds. This could push the wax into the ear canal and damage the ear drum. Instead, put a few drops of warm olive oil into the ear twice a week and the wax may soften and work itself free. There is a saying: 'the smallest thing you should put in your ear is your elbow'.

If you consult a doctor, he can remove the wax by syringing the ear, or remove any small hard lumps of wax with a probe.

It isn't true that ears can adjust to noise. Damage to the middle ear is irreparable. The level of noise should be reduced if it causes your ears to hurt or ring or if you have to shout to make yourself heard. If this is impossible, leave the source immediately.

Buy a good quality personal stereo to ensure you get a good reception with a low volume. Never wear headphones for longer than an hour at any given time. Limit time at rock concerts or clubs to two hours. Protect children's ears from loud explosions such as fireworks.

Always wear special ear protectors in a noisy working environment or when using power tools. If exposed to a high degree of constant noise, have periodic hearing checks. Always be aware that noise is not just irritating, it can also be a danger to your health.

Do not buy a hearing-aid without having a proper examination by your doctor. When there is pain, ringing in the ear or a discharge, or if you suspect that there may be a foreign body lodged inside, consult a doctor as soon as possible.

Ear-rings

For ear piercing, choose a jeweller or specialist beauty salon. There should be strictly hygienic conditions. Ear piercing should be painless as the ear lobes are lightly anaesthetised and the holes are made with a disposable needle attached to a syringe-shaped plunger.

Choose studs instead of ring 'sleepers' as the first ear-rings; they are less likely to get entangled in hair or clothes. Where possible choose gold earrings or at least gold posts as these are less likely to cause allergies.

Keep the first ear-rings in place for three months. They should be washed and turned twice daily. Some salons or jewellers prescribe an alcohol solution to clean around the ear-ring. Otherwise, clean the ear lobes with a warm saltwater solution.

Avoid fiddling with the ear-rings, and be careful they are not pulled out when undressing. If ear-rings are not worn for a long period of time the holes will close up.

Pretty Eyes

To test for satisfactory eyesight you should be able to read a car number plate at 23 m/80 ft. Eyesight should be checked regularly. Squinting to read or see something distant causes stress and wrinkles.

Good quality sun-glasses should be worn when sunbathing or driving in sunshine. Wear protective goggles when travelling on a motorcycle, welding or working with power tools.

When symptoms of redness, itching and swollen eyelids develop, it is probably a cosmetic allergy. Go without make-up until the symptoms disappear and do not use the product again.

Do not borrow or lend eye cosmetics as infections are easily passed from person to person. It is best to buy eye make-up from a reputable manufacturer. People with contact lenses usually require special hypo-allergenic make-up to avoid irritation.

Avoid putting on eye make-up when travelling as the eye can be accidentally poked with the brush or pencil. Always apply and remove mascara gently to avoid pulling out eyelashes.

When doing close-up work make sure there is adequate lighting. Natural lighting is best, but if a lamp is used, position it so that the light comes over the shoulder. Adjustable desk lamps will give a softer light than overhead fluorescent ones. Repair any flickering lights immediately.

Remember to blink frequently when concentrating hard. This is especially needed if wearing contact lenses. Rest the eyes periodically by looking into the distance. The further away you look the more relaxation is given to the eye muscle.

To relax and revitalise eye muscles when working as a VDU operator hold a pencil about 30 cm/1 ft away from the eyes, blink and focus on it.

You should see two VDU screens. Blink again and focus on the VDU screen; you will see two pencils.

Bring relief to tired eyes by sitting in a relaxed position, eyes closed and covered with slightly cupped hands. Rest elbows on cushions on the lap, relax and let the mind wander for 10 minutes.

Before going to bed, splash closed eyes 20 times with cold water then 20 times with warm. This technique can be applied during the day but use the warm water first. To revive tired eyes, apply fresh apple peel and rest for a few minutes.

Foreign Body in the Eye

One of the most common emergencies is caused by a foreign body in the eye. The tiniest speck of grit can cause immense discomfort and irritation. Do not rub the eye under any circumstances.

Sit the person on a chair facing the light and stand behind the chair, letting the head rest against you. Separate the lids of the affected eye and look for the foreign body. If it is in a very obvious position, remove with the dampened corner of a clean handkerchief, gauze or a moist cotton wool bud. It could also be flushed out with clean warm water or eye lotion.

If it is under the upper lid, grasp the lashes and pull the lid down over the lower lid. Do not poke the eye with any instruments. If you cannot remove the object, cover the eye with a clean pad, secure lightly and get medical help as soon as possible.

Eyebrow Grooming

Eyebrows perform the very important function of preventing sweat running into the eyes. Take the same trouble with the eyebrows as with the hair or eyelashes as they are a dominant facial feature and echo the shape of the eyes.

Groom eyebrows regularly, using an eyebrow brush or dry, clean toothbrush. Brush first against the direction of growth to remove any loose hairs and flakes of skin, then brush back into shape.

Any hairs growing across the bridge of the nose, or long stragglers under the brow can be removed with tweezers to neaten the shape.

To create a softer look, brush the brows upwards and use a little hair gel to keep them in place. Do not use hair spray as it could get into the eyes.

If eyebrows are too thin or patchy, fill them out – depending on your colouring – with dark brown or grey eyeshadow pencil or block mascara on a cotton wool bud. Do not use eyebrow pencil as it looks hard and unnatural.

When hair is lightened and the brows look too dark, they can be bleached to match. It is essential to have this done professionally. Never use depilatory creams or shave the eyebrows.

Before plucking, press cotton wool soaked in hot water on the area to open the pores. Using slant-tipped tweezers, hold the skin taut, grip each

individual hair with the tweezers and pull firmly in
the direction of growth. After you have finished
plucking, calm the irritated area with a splash of
cold water or a gentle skin toner.

Never remove hairs from the top of the brow, as
this arch delicately echoes the line of your eyes.

Do not reduce the width of the brows too much.
They should start at the point where the nose
meets the eye socket and continue beyond the
edge of the eye to a point that would make a
straight line with the corner of the mouth and
the outer edge of the eye.

If eyebrows have been plucked too severely,
disguise with eye-shadow as described above
and wear a sweatband when exercising.

Nosebleeds

Nosebleeds or epistaxis can be quite alarming. The
lining membrane of the nose has a rich supply of
tiny veins and if damaged, they bleed profusely.

Young children often have nosebleeds as
a result of 'picking' their nose. Soften any scabs or
crusts inside the nose with petroleum jelly; if
there is infection get your doctor to prescribe an
antibiotic cream. Children with allergies are
especially prone to nosebleeds as they tend to
sneeze and blow their nose more frequently.

Always get medical attention if a nosebleed occurs
after an accident or blow to the head.

To stop a nosebleed: sit the person on a chair with the head bent slightly forward over a bowl or sink. Loosen collar. Pinch the nose firmly, just below the hard part for at least ten minutes without releasing the pressure. Tell the patient to breathe through the mouth. Clench a cork or pad between the teeth to avoid the swallowing of blood, which disturbs clot formation and prolongs bleeding.

Wrap an ice cube in a tissue or cloth and place on the bridge of the nose to constrict the blood vessels and decrease the flow, thus allowing a clot to form. After releasing the nostrils, sit quietly. If bleeding restarts, squeeze the nostrils for a further ten minutes. Do not blow the nose for at least three hours.

Avoid taking alcohol or spicy foods and do not bend over or do any heavy manual work for 12 hours. If the bleeding cannot be stopped by the above measures, particularly in an elderly person, seek medical advice. Repeated nosebleeds may result in having to have a blood vessel cauterised by the doctor.

Dental Care

Plaque is the greatest cause of tooth decay and gum problems. It is a thin, colourless, sticky substance composed mainly of bacteria. Plaque forms almost continuously around the teeth and gums unless it is removed by regular brushing. A build-up of plaque hardens into a deposit called tartar on the teeth. This can be felt with the tongue and can only be removed by a dentist.

Sugary and starchy food interact with plaque on the teeth and produce acid. This acid attacks the tooth enamel and causes decay. The acidity can last up to two hours after a meal so the number of meals consumed is as relevant as the food eaten.

Limit sweet foods to mealtimes; other foods help to reduce the acid produced. At the end of a meal, if it is not convenient to brush your teeth, have a small piece of cheese to help neutralise the acid.

Although the saying goes 'an apple a day keeps the doctor away', this is not true for the dentist. Fruit such as apples help to produce acid in the mouth. People who suffer from a dry mouth may find it beneficial to chew sugar-free gum for a minimum of 20 minutes after a meal.

Brush the teeth regularly for about three minutes, especially after breakfast and at bedtime. Brushing gently with a small amount of baking soda or salt will help the teeth sparkle.

Replace a toothbrush when the head starts to lose its shape, or at least every three months. Choose one with the head small enough to reach every part of your mouth. Dentists recommend that a toothbrush should have medium to soft nylon bristles, a flat, even brushing surface, densely packed bristles, a straight handle and a medium to small head.

Waxed or unwaxed dental floss or tape is useful for dislodging trapped food and removing plaque from the crevices.

To floss teeth, take 60 cm/2 ft floss and wrap the ends around the middle fingers until you have around 7.5cm/3 in to work with. Hold the floss taut between the thumbs or index fingers to guide it between the teeth. Rub on both sides of each tooth using a new section of floss each time.

If gums tend to bleed, rinse the mouth with a saltwater solution. Report such problems to the dentist during your regular check-up.

To preserve a tooth knocked out in an accident: do not clean the tooth, use disinfectant on it or let it become dry. Immediately immerse the tooth in a cup of full-fat milk where it will keep for up to 12 hours, allowing time to visit the dentist to have it reinserted.

It is vital to have the tooth replaced in the socket as quickly as possible, since the nerve endings tend to die and the socket begins to heal., causing the reinsertion to be unsuccessful.

Beautiful Breasts

A well-fitting bra is very important. If it is too loose it will not support the breasts; a tight bra will rub against the skin and be uncomfortable.

Always wear a bra when exercising or playing sport. There are special sports bras that are made from soft cotton and are seamless across the nipples to prevent friction. Some sports bras have no cups and are like short vests that bind the breasts close to the chest.

To work out bra measurements: for the back size, wearing a bra and standing straight, measure under the bust and add 10 cm/4 in. It may be easier to get someone to help you.

To find the cup size: measure the fullest part of the bust. Then measure above the bust. The difference between these measurements gives the cup size. The sizes are as follows: size A, a difference between 1 cm/½ in and 4 cm/1½ in; size B, between 4 cm/1½ in and 6 cm/2½ in; size C, between 6 cm/2½ in and 9 cm/3½ in; size D, between 9 cm/3½ in and 12 cm/4¼ in.

Check that the cup completely covers the breast. Bulges at the top or sides indicate that the cup is too small. Neither should the sides of the cup wrinkle because the breast does not fill it.

The bra should be snug but not tight around the body. If it is cutting into your flesh, the back size is too small or the back closure should be hooked less tightly. The back of the bra should stay down on the body. If it slips up then the bra size may be too large, it may be hooked too loosely or the straps may be adjusted too tightly. The centre of the bra should lie against the breast bone. If it stretches away from the body, the cup size is too small.

The straps should be adjusted to support the breasts comfortably without pressure. Check the width of the strap for your personal preference.

The only possible ways to achieve a smaller bust are surgery or aerobic exercises which burn fatty tissue from all over the body. Disregard creams or miracle cures as they are ineffective.

Every woman should check her breasts regularly for lumps. This should be done at the same time every month, a few days after her period. Self-checking is often taught at local clinics or your doctor will show you the correct method.

Stand before a mirror with your hands above your head and look at your breasts closely for puckering or any visible changes.

Lie down on a towel on the floor, hunch up the left shoulder. Feel carefully for any lumps or other unusual signs at the top of the left breast.

Raise your arm above your head and continue to feel around the whole breast. Use your fingers rather than the palm of your hand. Check into the armpit area. Repeat this with the right breast.

If you notice any change or feel any unusual lumps go and see your general practitioner immediately. Most lumps are benign but, if not, early diagnosis minimises the treatment.

Tummy Troubles

Effective chewing is important for digestion so only put small amounts of food into the mouth. Eat slowly and really taste the food, chewing with the mouth closed. Learn to relax when eating by putting the knife and fork down occasionally, and take smaller mouthfuls rather than gulping food.

A glass of wine with a meal is relaxing and will aid digestion. Have a short rest after a meal to allow the food to be digested more effectively.

Take small meals at regular intervals. The stomach is constantly producing acid. Irregular meals mean the acid has long periods with no food to digest and this causes 'heartburn', or indigestion.

Have regular exercise daily – even a short walk. Avoid foods you know, though experience, will upset your stomach. Smoking, alcohol, drugs such as aspirin, coffee and tea can irritate the stomach lining. After a course of antibiotics, eat a yogurt daily to renew stomach enzymes and avoid indigestion.

To avoid insomnia, do not overeat. Supper should be several hours before bedtime. To relieve night-time indigestion, raise the head of the bed about 10 cm/4 inches. Antacid medicine or sips of soda water will help relieve symptoms but if constantly bothered with indigestion or worried about frequent stomach pains it is advisable to visit the doctor.

Hard-working Hands

For hygienic reasons hands should be kept clean and as germ-free as possible.

When washing hands remove all rings, use warm water and a little soap. Rinse them well and dry thoroughly, especially between the fingers. Apply a barrier cream to hands before commencing chores

Wear plastic or rubber gloves when working with chemical products such as detergents, white spirit, turpentine, dry-cleaning fluid or petrol.

Rich hand creams will be more effective if used at night and the hands covered with a pair of cotton gloves. Lighter creams may be applied frequently during the day. When applying hand creams, always massage the hands well.

Remove stains on hands by rubbing them with the inside skin of a lemon or orange, or a potato slice.

To remove tough stains on the palms of the hands, try massaging them with 5 ml/10 tsp sea-salt or granulated sugar mixed with a few drops of olive or vegetable oil. Rinse, dry well and moisturise.

A natural hand cream: combine to a smooth paste 15 ml/1 tbsp honey, 30 ml/2 tbsp ground almonds and an egg yolk. Apply to the hands and leave on for 15 minutes. Rinse off and dry well. Rub a little homemade mayonnaise thoroughly into your hands and wipe away any surplus.

Neat Nails

Avoid nails breaking by keeping them fairly short, especially when using a typewriter. Never use nails to prise open compacts, untie laces or string.

Cutting nails with scissors will weaken the nail so use a nail file or emery board. File one way only from side to centre. Back and forth rubbing shreds the nail fibres and causes splitting.

Always use proper enamel remover and refrain from peeling off old enamel as a layer of nail can also come off. Never use neat acetone to remove varnish; it will dry and split the nails. Cosmetic removers have special oils added to prevent nail damage.

Leave nails free of nail varnish occasionally. Constant use, especially without a base-coat, can cause yellowing of the nails.

An excellent nail conditioner is a soak for 10 minutes in hot oil. Try either hot almond, castor, wheatgerm or baby oil.

Massaging or buffing nails improves circulation and stimulates growth. Buff nails with a little almond oil or beeswax on a soft, closely woven, natural cloth wrapped around a ball of cotton wool, or with a buffer, a soft pad covered in fine leather.

Next, apply a moisturising nail cream: mix together 5 ml/1 tsp each avocado, liquid honey and egg yolk. Rub into and around the finger nails. Rinse off after half an hour.

Gently push back the cuticles with a soft cloth when washing the hands. Rub cuticles with hand cream or special cuticle cream. Never cut or dig under a cuticle.

Cuticle cream: mix 30ml/2 tbsp each pineapple juice and egg yolk with 2.5 ml/½ tsp cider vinegar. Soak the nails in this for half an hour and then rinse off. Use nightly to 'feed' the growing nails.

Discoloured nails: always apply a colourless base coat before varnish. Avoid continuous use of nail varnish and refrain from smoking.

To remove stains, rub with lemon juice followed by white wine vinegar, then massage with almond oil.

DID YOU KNOW?
White flecks or 'chalk marks' on the nails are just immature cells which didn't become transparent. It has nothing to do with lack of calcium. They can be more prevalent after injury to a nail or after manicuring. It takes five months for a complete nail to grow and it grows more quickly during the summer months. Nails also grow more quickly on the hand you use most, and on the longer fingers.

Pampering Your Feet

Every day, especially if the feet are tired and aching, lie down, elevate the feet and massage the legs from foot to knee. This relieves pressure and improves the circulation.

To stimulate circulation give feet a good daily scrub in warm water. Rub down dry skin with a pumice stone. Don't soak feet for longer than 10 minutes as the natural oils will tend to dry out.

Add a handful of Epsom salts or baking soda with a few drops lavender oil for a special treat. A dash of added cider vinegar will help eliminate itching and prevent athlete's foot.

Dry well, especially between the toes, and use surgical spirit rather than talcum powder. Manicure the toe nails when the skin is soft after washing. Cut toe nails straight across to strengthen them and discourage ingrown toe nails.

When hard nails are difficult to cut, dab the nail with a piece of cotton wool soaked in peroxide and leave it on for a few minutes.

Every night rub glycerine or moisturising cream on any dry skin on the feet, especially the heels and toe joints, where hard skin is prone to develop. Buy sensible shoes, choose the style carefully and have them properly fitted. They should fit closely at the heel with plenty of toe room.

Foot Complaints

Athlete's foot (*tinea pedis*) is a fungal infection causing cracked, red and itchy skin between the toes. It thrives in warm, moist conditions and is exacerbated by sweat or not thoroughly drying the foot after washing. It can spread to the sole of the foot. To clear up the infection, powder and cream can be purchased in a chemist's shop. To prevent recurrence, wear cotton socks, use a selection of shoes, dry between toes carefully and do not walk barefoot at public swimming pools. Sometimes the fungus can lie dormant and break out repeatedly. Your doctor can prescribe antibiotics in this case.

Calluses are found mainly on the ball and heel of the foot. They are areas of hard thick skin caused by badly fitted shoes. Remove the dead skin with a pumice stone or special skin removing cream but use with care so that the skin is not broken. To prevent calluses, moisturise feet frequently.

Chilblains are shiny red swellings on the toes. They are caused by poor circulation from standing outdoors in the cold. When the feet warm up they become painful and itchy. Avoid scratching or the skin will break and become infected. Calamine lotion will help soothe the irritation.

For chilblains: mix 15 ml/1 tbsp honey with equal glycerine, the white of one egg and enough flour to make a fine paste. Add 5 ml/1 tsp rose water if required. Apply to chilblains and cover with cotton cloth.

Other age-old cures are bathing them frequently in your own fresh urine or rubbing them with a slice of onion dipped in salt. To prevent chilblains, wear warm socks and well-insulated shoes. Exercise legs and feet as well to increase blood circulation. Do not warm the feet directly in front of the fire or on a hot water bottle.

Hammer toes usually affect the second or third toe. The toes are bent downwards and sometimes calluses form on them. They are caused by short narrow shoes or tight socks. The first corrective measure is to have properly fitted footwear. A chiropodist can provide padding for the toes but if the damage is severe, surgery may be necessary.

Ingrown toe nails dig into the flesh at either side of the toe and can be very painful. The big toe is usually the one affected. Sometimes the surrounding area is red and swollen and the nail may even cut into it.

If the area is infected then consult a doctor but otherwise treat by soaking the foot in warm water for 10 minutes. Then with a nail file lift the ingrown part of the nail and slip a piece of cotton wool under it. Remove and replace with fresh cotton wool daily until the nail grows beyond the corner of the toe. To avoid ingrown toe nails cut the nail straight across. Do not wear narrow or pointed shoes that crush the toes.

Corns are hard lumps of thick dead skin. They are generally found on the top or the side of the toes where they rub against the shoes. If they hurt, soak the foot in warm soapy water for 10 minutes. Rub the corn with an emery board twice a week after soaking. You can purchase special corn plasters that will prevent the shoe irritating the corn. Never cut a corn with a razor blade as you may get it infected. Ask a chiropodist to trim it using sterilised instruments.

Bunions are growths over the bone at the first joint of the big toes. Since there is a dislocation of the joint the big toe may be tight against the second toe or even overlapping it. Tight narrow shoes aggravate bunions and they can be very painful. Avoid wearing high-heeled narrow shoes and whenever possible go barefoot. Pads to separate the toes and reduce the pressure can be purchased at chemists. In severe cases, surgery involving the reconstruction of the toe joint will probably be recommended by your doctor or chiropodist. Bunions tend to be hereditary.

Pain at the back of the heel is usually caused by changing from high heels to flats or bare feet. This can cause the cordlike Achilles tendon at the back of the heel to overstretch. Sometimes the pain runs right up the leg to the back of the knee. For relief, apply an ice-pack for ten minutes.

To avoid further damage do this calf-stretching exercise for two minutes every day for two weeks: standing barefoot, place the palms of the hands against the wall and stand at arm's length. Keeping the back straight and feet flat on the floor, bend your arms until your nose touches the wall. Push back slowly and repeat.

Painful balls of the feet can be caused by high heels as these throw the weight forward, putting pressure on the metatarsus. Other causes are high arches or prominent metatarsal bones. To ease the pain, apply an ice-pack or bathe in cold running water. Wear shoes with flat heels and check with your chemist or chiropodist for special insoles or pads that will help relieve the pressure.

Fallen arches or 'flat feet' can be caused by bad posture. They cause the foot to roll inwards at the ankle, making them ache, and sometimes also cause back pain.

A chiropodist can fit an arch support in the shoe and prescribe strengthening exercises. In severe cases surgery may be needed.

Foot odour occurs when the feet are warm and moist and the sweat cannot evaporate. It can be more prevalent during puberty because of changes in hormone levels.

To reduce the problem, wear cotton or wool socks which absorb the sweat. Wash the feet frequently in warm water, rinse in cool or cold water and dry well, then wipe with surgical spirit. Use foot and shoe antiperspirant, deodorant sprays or powders, or special shoe insoles that absorb sweat. If possible change your tights, socks and shoes daily. Wear shoes made of skin or leather, including the soles. Whenever possible, wear sandals or go barefoot.

Tired feet: soak the feet in a basin of warm water containing a handful of salt for about 10 minutes. Wriggle the toes to relieve the cramping effect of shoes. Dry the feet, lie on your back and put your feet up against a wall for 15 minutes.

For a herbal footbath: add a handful each of dried thyme and peppermint leaves to 600 ml/1 pint water. Bring to the boil and simmer for 5 minutes. Add enough cold water to cool to a comfortable temperature. Soak the feet in this for 10 minutes. Alternatively, pour 600 ml/1 pint boiling water over 30 ml/2 tbsp fresh nettle leaves and flowers. Leave to infuse for two or three hours. Warm the solution and soak the feet for at least five minutes.

A verruca is a painful viral wart that has grown inwards from the pressure of standing. A layer of skin can grow over the verruca. It should be covered when attending the public swimming pool.

Consult a chiropodist for removal, which may be surgical removal by freezing or burning, or creams or ointment may be applied and the wart scraped away slowly over a period of weeks.

DID YOU KNOW?
The foot has 26 delicate bones held together with muscle and ligaments. By the age of 70, our feet will probably have carried us the equivalent of three times around the world.

Salutary Skin

Care of the skin begins with a healthy diet with adequate vitamins, and the elimination of stress. Exercise and adequate sleep both play their part. The skin surface can be covered with flaking dead skin, excreted toxins and grime. Removing these from the skin and keeping it clean and fresh is a very important part of good skin care.

Skin should be cleansed regularly, have sufficient moisture and always be protected from strong sun. Soap and water is an effective skin cleanser but it is alkaline and can upset the natural acid balance of the skin, pH 4.5- 5.5. Sometimes this causes dryness and the skin reacts by producing more oil, the result being greasy skin. Choose soaps with nearly the same pH balance as skin, or use cream cleansers and lotions, which are very efficient for removing make-up and grime.

Before bathing use a body scrub to improve the circulation and remove dead skin cells, thereby smoothing the skin. Use a loofah or try a scrub of sea-salt or oatmeal. Granulated sugar mixed with oil is ideal for rubbing on elbows, knees or feet.

To nourish the skin, fill a muslin bag with bran or oatmeal and soak it in the bath by hanging it from the tap so it can be used several times.

To counteract skin dryness, add oil to the bath. The floating oil clings to the skin and lubricates it. To relieve tiredness add 15 ml/1 tbsp honey. For luxury add a handful of powdered milk or fill a muslin bag with herbs and suspend it in the water.

Body odour: soap and water may not be sufficient. In this case use a deodorant or antiperspirant. A deodorant masks odour and inhibits bacterial growth but does not affect the flow of perspiration.

An antiperspirant is composed of chemicals which partially block the pores and reduce the perspiration reaching the skin's surface. Use antiperspirants sparingly since perspiration helps regulate the body temperature.

Natural deodorant: use green leaves, fresh green vegetables such as beet tops or spinach, fresh herbs such as mint. Rub the leaves briskly over problem areas during the day. Alternatively shake six drops lavender oil in 600 ml/1 pint distilled water. Store in fridge. Apply with cotton wool twice daily.

Body lotion for dry skin: combine 30 ml/2 tbsp lime juice, 45 ml/3 tbsp rose water and 15 ml/ 1 tbsp glycerine until the mixture is smooth.

Sensitive skin reacts adversely to some external influences. The usual cause is cosmetic ingredients but temperature extremes or poor skin care can also be cited. Symptoms vary from dry, flaking skin, rashes, itching, blotches, reddening and even painful swelling. There are two separate problems: irritation and allergy. They show similar skin reactions but have different causes.

Irritation is the most common problem. The skin type most prone is usually fair and dry. It is caused by strong detergents, harsh products containing alcohol, using the wrong products for the skin type or sometimes hot water or cold winds. A reaction occurs immediately or very soon afterwards and worsens if large amounts of the product is applied. The cure is to avoid harsh products. Use baby products or cleansing milk. Never use very hot or cold water, only lukewarm.

An allergy occurs when the body reacts to a substance which it thinks is harmful. The auto-immune system goes into action and sends white blood cells rushing to the skin's surface. This makes the skin red, itchy and sore. The reaction can take up to a week to appear and sometimes a product can cause an allergy after years of use. However once the skin has an allergic reaction to a product or substance, it will stay this way for ever. Allergies can occur with any skin type.

To cure an allergy, first find the cause. A new cosmetic product is an obvious choice, otherwise all products in use will have to be removed in turn to find the problem. A food allergy can also cause a

skin reaction so the diet may have to be checked.
When the problem product is found a doctor can
do patch tests on the skin with each ingredient to
determine which one is causing the reaction. For
products used over a long time, but now causing a
reaction, it may be worthwhile contacting the
manufacturers to ascertain if they have changed
the composition of the product.

Spotty Problems

Many teenagers suffer from acne or inflamed spots.
These result from a bacterial infection causing
inflammation around a sebaceous gland, and can
occur on the back and chest as well as the face.
Although it cannot be prevented, it can be
controlled. Medical preparations are available from
chemists but in severe cases special treatment from
a doctor will be required.

When suffering from acne, seek medical advice
at an early stage and use the prescribed treatment
for the recommended time. Avoid changing
treatments if results are not showing in a short
time. Most treatments take three months to work
and some antibiotic courses can last for six months.
It is vital to keep the skin clean using good quality
products, but very frequent washing can aggravate
the problem. Avoid squeezing spots as this can
cause scarring. It is a myth that chocolate and fatty
food cause acne or make it worse.

For acne: drink three cups freshly brewed nettle
tea daily before meals. Pour 250 ml/8 fl oz boiling
water over 6 ml/1 heaped tbsp chopped nettle

leaves. Cover and leave for two minutes. Strain and sip slowly.

To calm a spot: mix 5 ml/1 tsp lemon juice with 5 ml/1 tsp salt and apply. Leave for 10 minutes and rinse off. To disguise a spot, dab with calamine lotion before applying foundation or colour it with an eyebrow pencil for an instant beauty mark.

Sunbathing

A good tan must be acquired slowly. Do not stay in the sun more than half an hour the first day. Increase the length of time daily. The depth of the tan reaches a maximum after eight days. More sunbathing just produces dry, peeling skin. People with pale complexions should avoid the midday sun.

When walking to the beach remember you are out in the sunshine so apply sunscreen before starting off. Be careful where you sunbathe – sand and concrete surfaces can reflect the sun back at you, causing the skin to burn more easily.

Use waterproof sunscreen when swimming as the body will still catch the sun. Reapply hourly to maintain adequate protection.

Most sunscreen products have a sun protection factor (SPF) rating on them. Generally, people with pale blue or green eyes need a strong factor, while those with hazel or brown eyes need less. Some medical research has shown that while both men and women with dark brown eyes were least at risk, men with dark blue eyes and women with pale blue eyes were most vulnerable.

Children should wear light clothing as well as a sunscreen. It can take up to four hours for sunburn to show on the skin so don't be fooled by the pale skin colour. A haze or a light covering of cloud over the sun does not stop ultra-violet rays from coming through and causing burning. Use a higher sun protection factor on the face, shoulders, ankles and feet as these areas are very easily burned.

The best way to get an even tan is to keep moving – go for walks, play games, or do the gardening. Sun dries out the skin so use after-sun products to lock in moisture and reduce skin peeling. Sun-bed treatment before sunbathing does not prevent sunburn. Like the sun, sun-beds will accelerate skin ageing and increase the chance of skin cancer.

If you do get sunburn, the skin will be red, feeling tight and sore. In this case, cool the body with a long tepid shower. Soothe the skin with calamine lotion or plain yogurt.

Alternatively, combine 15 ml/1 tbsp olive oil and 15 ml/1 tbsp glycerine. Add two drops eucalyptus oil and smear gently over the affected area, or wipe the skin with cotton wool soaked in cooled camomile tea.

There are many fake tan preparations on the market which create a natural, healthy effect. However, these do not protect skin from the sun.

Home-Grown Beauty Treatments

Homemade Preparations

For years natural things like petals, herbs, leaves, roots, fruit and vegetables have been used to make beauty preparations. Make your own concoctions.

Success with homemade beauty treatments will depend on whether the skin is suitable for the recipe, so always do a patch test in case of an allergic reaction to the ingredients. It is generally best to make only enough mixture for one application and use it immediately. Some recipes can be used for a few applications but remember that homemade mixtures contain no stabilisers or preservatives so only make up small quantities and store in the fridge.

Unless otherwise stated, discard all preparations after four days. Use stainless steel or enamel containers to prepare treatments. Avoid non-stick or aluminium as these may alter the nature of the preparation. Sterilise the storage jars or bottles you use. If the potion becomes infected with bacteria it will go off quickly and can cause illness.

Date and label the jars. Glass jars and bottles are the best containers as metal may taint the potion. The lids should be screw-top and airtight. Always use fresh ingredients and measure them carefully as accuracy will produce more successful results.

Before applying any preparation, cleanse the face. Use a shower cap, hair band or clips to keep hair out of the way if necessary.

Using Fruit and Vegetables

Masks should be left on for 15-20 minutes so they can dry. Rinse off with lots of tepid water. If you feel that any treatment is irritating your skin, wipe off immediately and rinse well with tepid water. All mask pastes should be of a consistency that is easy to smooth onto the face without dragging. Apply paste with clean fingertips or a soft brush. If lotions or masks are very slushy, place a piece of muslin or gauze on the face to keep them in place.

Choose a time to use masks or lotions when you know you are not going to be disturbed and can relax. Wash all the ingredients before use and discard any that are damaged. An electric blender or liquidiser will make the mixing easier.

Avocado: has a high oil content and is rich and nourishing for the skin. A dry or sensitive face, hands or nails will benefit from a mask made from the pulp, which should be quite ripe. Skin half an avocado and mash with 20 ml/1 tbsp tomato pulp and 15 ml/1 tbsp lemon juice. Spread over the face and neck and relax for 20 minutes. Rinse off with tepid water and pat skin dry. Suits all types of skin. For dry skin: mash a ripe avocado until smooth, add 5 ml/1 tsp both lemon juice and honey. Mix to a paste. Apply over the face and neck, avoiding the eye areas. This mixture can also applied to dry hair before washing to restore lustre.

Banana: a moisturising face mask for all skin types. Mash a large banana, mix in 5 ml/1 tsp each milk, cream and honey. Add one vitamin E capsule. Apply to the face and neck. Leave for 20 minutes and rinse off with warm water.

Carrot: liquidise carrot to a pulp and use as a mask for cleansing the skin. This can be used on all skin types and is especially good for sensitive skin. As a cleanser, put 45 ml/3 tbsp finely grated carrot and 45 ml/3 tbsp finely chopped spinach leaves into a bowl and immerse in 100 ml/7 tbsp boiling water. Cover and infuse for eight hours. Add 200 ml/ 14 tbsp milk, beat well and leave for a further two hours. Strain, bottle and store in the fridge.

Cucumber: as a face pack, mash 50 g/2 oz peeled cucumber with 10 ml/2 tsp powdered milk and one whisked egg white. For dry skin, mash half a cucumber with a small carton cold, natural yogurt. Leave on for 30 minutes, rinse off and moisturise.

For greasy skin: blend half a peeled cucumber to a pulp, add 2.5 ml/½ tsp lemon juice, 5ml/1 tsp witch hazel and one whisked egg white.

For all skin types: add 15 ml/1 tbsp cucumber or tomato pulp to 15 ml/1 tbsp natural yogurt. Leave on skin for 10-15 minutes and wash off with warm water. Pat dry. Use cucumber slices to soothe puffy or tired eyes. Soothe sunburnt skin with a paste of mashed cucumber.

Green pepper: liquidise and add to any of your favourite face masks to soften the skin.

Lemon: rub 'empty' lemon halves on dull or hard skin, especially elbows, to soften, clean and bleach. Comb pure lemon juice through hair to lighten. To alleviate greasiness add a dash to the rinsing water. For greasy skin, mix an egg white with an equal amount of lemon juice and 125 ml/4 fl oz water. Spread this over the skin and rinse off after five minutes.

'Sugaring' to remove unwanted body hair: put 125 ml/¼ pint lemon juice and 450 g/1 lb sugar into a saucepan. Heat slowly until the sugar has melted. Boil rapidly for a few minutes until caramel coloured. Pour into a warm, sterilised jar and cool. Apply a layer of the mixture to the skin, smooth on a strip of linen, press down, then quickly pull the strip off, going against the direction of the hair.

Lettuce: cover a handful of lettuce leaves with boiling water. Cool and strain; use as a toner.

Conditioning face mask: cook eight washed lettuce leaves in 300 ml/½ pint milk for three minutes or until soft but whole. Strain off the liquid and reserve. Place the warm leaves on clean face and gently press down. Relax for 20 minutes, then remove the leaves and rinse the skin with the reserved milk.

Melon: use chilled segments to soothe puffy eyes. Rub a slice of melon over the face to freshen the skin; soak a pad of cotton wool in the strained juice from a slice of mashed melon and use as a refreshing toner.

Melon and peach: mash together a slice of melon and half a peach for a face pack. Leave on the face for 10 minutes before rinsing off.

Mint and apple: this astringent toner should not be used on sensitive skin. Place 15 ml/1 tbsp chopped mint in a jar and add 30 ml/2 tbsp cider vinegar. Shake well and leave in the fridge for a few days. Strain the liquid and add 300 ml/½ pint water. Dab onto the skin with cotton wool.

Orange: mix ground dried orange peel with ground oatmeal and enough water to make a thick paste. Use as a face and body scrub.

Orange skin fresheners: wash, slice and score the peel of three oranges and place in a pan with 1.8 litres/3 pints boiling water. Cool, strain and use daily. Alternatively, pour the juice of ½ orange and ¼ lemon into a saucepan with 5 ml/1 tsp castor sugar and 250 ml/8 fl oz milk. Heat to near boiling point and leave to cool before use. Refreshing orange mask for all skin types: heat 45 ml/3 tbsp honey and the juice of ½ orange over a low flame until just warm. Pat onto the face.

Peach: mash a peach or apricot to a pulp. Add 5 ml/1 tsp honey and 30 ml/2 tbsp powdered milk and stir well. Leave on the face for 30 minutes.

Potato: use potato water as a cleanser for oily skin. Refresh normal skin with raw potato or lime slices.

Strawberry: for a toner for sensitive skin or to calm sunburn, mash strawberries and apply for

5 minutes as a soothing mask, or mash two large strawberries with 15 ml/1 tbsp yogurt or cream. Smooth onto the face and leave for 10 minutes.

Alternatively, blend 100 g/4 oz fresh or defrosted strawberries with half a lemon. Add 30 ml/2 tbsp cream to form a paste. Avoiding the eyes, apply mixture with a brush and leave on the face for at least an hour. If strawberries are unavailable try using tomato flesh.

For a strawberry skin cleanser, mash three large strawberries to a pulp, add 300 ml/½ pint milk and whisk thoroughly. Apply to the skin and leave to dry. This suits all skin.

Tomato: as an astringent, pulp a tomato and pat onto the skin. To cleanse the back, sieve or liquidise two soft tomatoes and combine with one carton natural yogurt. Smooth this mixture over the back and leave for 20 minutes, then rinse.

Using Shoots and Roots

Roots, herbs and leaves may be used thus:
An **infusion** is just a strong 'tea'. Pour 250 ml/ 8 fl oz boiling water over 5 ml/1 tsp dried or 10 ml/2 tsp fresh herbs. Leave for 10-15 minutes. Strain and drink hot or cold three times a day.

Decoction is the extraction of the essences of roots and seeds by boiling. Use the same proportions as for infusion but add a little extra water to allow for evaporation. Simmer for 30 minutes. Strain, cool and drink one cup three times daily.

Massage oils can be made by gently heating 150 ml/¼ pint olive or vegetable oil with 5ml/1 tsp preferred herb, until it starts to discolour. Remove immediately from the heat and leave to cool. Strain the mixture well and use it for for massaging the body after a bath.

A **compress** is a wad of cotton wool dipped in a warm herbal infusion or decoction.

Herbal baths: heat 600ml/1 pint cider vinegar and 600 ml/1 pint water but do not boil. Add 90 ml/ 6 tbsp chopped mixed herbs such as elderflower, eucalyptus, lemon balm, mint and simmer for 10 minutes. Strain and add to the bath water for a refreshing bath.

A **tincture** is a herbal extract preserved in alcohol. Cover 100 g/3 ½ oz freshly chopped or dried herbs with 500 ml/17 fl oz vodka in a wide-rimmed jar and seal it. Store in a cool dark place and shake daily. After 2 weeks, strain and decant into a dark bottle. Take 5-10 drops three times daily added to water, tea or fruit juice, as preferred.

Some suggestions for extractions: cinnamon to stimulate the appetite; cloves to soothe toothache; dandelion to brighten dull skin; garlic to relieve catarrh and improve digestion; marigold to help clear skin, especially oily; mint to freshen breath; parsley to help eliminate scurf or darken hair; rhubarb root to highlight mousy hair; rosemary to refresh the feet; sage to close pores and darken grey hair; thyme as an invigorating scalp tonic.

Refreshing herbal bath: heat 600 ml/1 pint cider vinegar and 600 ml/1 pint water, but do not boil. Add 90 ml/6 tbsp chopped mixed herbs, such as elderflower, eucalyptus, lemon balm, mint, and simmer for 10 minutes. Strain; add to bath water.

To soothe under-eye puffiness: boil a handful of chopped rosehips in 300 ml/½ pint water for 10 minutes. When just warm, soak two pads of cotton wool and cover eyes with them for 15 minutes.

Facial steam bath: do not use this treatment if you have sensitive skin or thread veins on your face. Pour 600 ml/1 pint boiling water over a handful of any mixed dried herbs in a large bowl. Keep covered while cleansing the face thoroughly. Drape a towel loosely over the head and holding the face at least 22 cm/9 inches above the water, steam for 5-10 minutes. Pat dry and wipe over with lotion.

Parsley face pack: boil a handful of fresh parsley in 300 ml/½ pint water for 10 minutes. Strain and cool, mix with 15 ml/1 tbsp honey and a stiffly beaten egg-white. Leave on face for 15-20 minutes.

Mud pack: pour 250 ml/8 fl oz boiling water over 30 ml/2 tbsp dried sage and parsley. Strain after 10 minutes. Take 15 ml/1 tbsp of this and mix with a whisked egg white. Add enough Fuller's Earth or kaolin to make a paste and use in the normal way.

Blackberry leaf: collect leaves from an area free from chemical pollutants. Make an infusion with a handful of crushed leaves in 300 ml/½ pint boiling water. Strain after an hour or when cool.

Use all the infusion for several nights in the bath to revitalise dry skin.

Raspberry leaf skin cleanser: prepare an infusion as for blackberry leaves. Apply 150 ml/¼ pint of the infusion mixed with 150 ml/¼ pint plain yogurt, then moisturise as usual.

Lotion for greasy skin: make an infusion of either lavender, lemon balm, rosemary or yarrow. Mix 150 ml/¼ pint of the cool, strained infusion with 150 ml/¼ pint natural yogurt.

Lotion for normal and dry skin: soak 45 ml/3 tbsp camomile, elderflower or meadowsweet in 300 ml/ ½ pint fresh milk for an hour. Heat almost to boiling, cool, strain, bottle, and store in the fridge.

Toner for greasy skin: pour 150 ml/¼ pint boiling water over 30 ml/2 tbsp chopped sage and allow to cool. Strain into 150 ml/¼ pint cider vinegar.

Toner for normal and dry skin: soak 30 ml/2 tbsp dried elderflower, meadowsweet, marshmallow or marigold in 600 ml/1 pint boiling water. Cover and leave to cool for one hour. Strain, bottle and cap.

Using Petals
Aromatic floral oils are extracted from petals. It takes hundreds of leaves to produce a few drops so they are expensive to produce. However only a few drops need be used to promote general well-being. There are three main ways of using the oils:
In the bath: make sure the bathroom is warm and

the doors and windows closed. Add a few drops of oil to the bath water and soak the body for 10 minutes; breathe deeply to inhale the vapours.

Massage: this is a very effective method for the oil to be absorbed into the body. Dilute the aromatic oil with almond oil to avoid causing irritation to the skin. Massage the body for at least 10 minutes.

Inhalation: add a few drops to a bowl of hot water. Put a towel over your head and lean over the bowl about 23 cm/9 inches above the water. Breathe deeply to inhale the vapours.

This method is not advisable for people who have sensitive skin, since the steam may cause broken veins and extreme redness of the complexion.

Some of the more common aromatic oils are:
Aloe Vera: soothes and heals burns and skin lesions. Commonly found in suntan preparations

Evening Primrose: may aid some pre-menstrual problems and various skin conditions

Lavender: beneficial for acne, bruising, dermatitis; also reduces swelling and heals burns

Rose: an excellent skin tonic. Make rose water by mixing 15 ml/1 tbsp rose oil with 2.25 litres/4 pints purified water. Bottle and store in the fridge

Ylang Ylang: this oil is useful as an antiseptic and tonic for the nervous system

Add 4-6 drops to a bath or 4 drops to 10 ml/2 tsp soya oil and use as a perfume

TONERS:
Combination skin: refresh the skin by mixing two parts of rose-water with one part of witch hazel and apply to the skin with cotton wool.

Dry skin: combine 30 ml/2 tbsp lemon juice, 15 ml/1 tbsp glycerine and 45 ml/3 tbsp rose water. Rub into the skin.

Oily skin: dissolve 5 ml/1 tsp borax in 150 ml/ ¼ pint rose water. Warm 30 ml/2 tbsp olive oil and slowly add to the mixture, beat with an egg whisk until it is thick and creamy. Add 30ml/2 tbsp lavender water.

General skin tonic: infuse a handful of dandelion flowers in 300 ml/½ pint boiling water, add 30 ml/ 2 tbsp dried thyme leaves and leave to cool for 20 minutes. Strain through a sieve and add 5 ml/ 1 tbsp witch hazel.

Soothing tonic: infuse 45 ml/3 tbsp dried or fresh marigold leaves in a bowl with 600 ml/1 pint boiling water for 20 minutes. Add 15 ml/1 tbsp apple juice and apply with cotton wool.

Place a **herbal pillow** either inside or under your bed pillow to give a soft fragrance to your bedroom and help you relax or induce sleep. The cover should be of thinly woven cotton. Use dried herbs as the aroma lasts longer. For relaxing: camomile, dill, geranium, lavender, lemon balm, mint, rose, rosemary, sage and thyme For inducing sleep: use mixed lavender and thyme with a pinch of dried grated orange peel and a shake of cinnamon.

Using Eggs, Honey and Oils

Oily skin mask: use a beaten egg white mixed with 1.25 ml/¼ tsp lemon juice or cider vinegar. Honey mask: make with 30 ml/2 tbsp honey mixed with 2.5 ml/½ tsp lemon juice or cider vinegar.

Normal skin: add 75 g/3 oz ground almonds to a 150 ml/¼ pint milk and mix well. Simmer until the liquid is absorbed; add a beaten egg yolk. Reheat until boiling then add 15 ml/1 tbsp almond oil. Cool and use before a bath as a body massage.

Dry skin: beat an egg yolk with 5 ml/1 tsp pure honey and smooth into the face and throat. If skin is very dry, a few drops of almond oil can be added to the mixture.

Sallow skin: if your skin feels dull, beat an egg yolk and mix with a little almond oil. Smooth over the face, leave for 10 minutes, remove with cotton wool and warm water.

Egg face pack: beat an egg white lightly then add a few drops of almond oil. Smooth over face and throat, avoiding the eye area, and leave until it firms slightly. Remove gently with warm water.

Use a moisturiser before your make-up. This face pack is suitable for dry and normal skin.

Nourishing face mask: mash the flesh of ½ ripe avocado pear, add a beaten egg white and 5 ml/ 1 tsp lemon juice. Whisk well, smooth over the face and throat and leave for 20 minutes. Remove with a face flannel and warm water.

Refining face mask: mix 15 ml/1 tbsp fine oatmeal, 5 ml/1 tsp lemon juice, a beaten egg white and enough yogurt to make a manageable mixture. Cover the face with a piece of gauze and spread the mixture over it. Leave on the face for 15-20 minutes. Remove gauze and wash face.

Face mask for regular use: beat an egg, 15 ml/ 1 tbsp milk, and 5 ml/1 tsp pure honey together and smooth over the face and throat. Leave for 15 minutes. Wash off with warm water and then splash face with tepid water.

Yogurt and egg face mask: beat the white of an egg until stiff and fold in 15 ml/1 tbsp yogurt.

Optional extras: add 5 ml/1 tsp honey for dry skin or 5 ml/1 tsp lemon juice for combination skin. Leave on for 10-15 minutes then rinse off with warm water.

Honey and cream face mask: beat together 5 ml/ 1 tsp honey with 30 ml/2 tbsp light cream. Leave on the face for 20 minutes.

To soften skin and relieve tension: take 125ml/ 8 fl oz almond oil, 125 ml/4 fl oz castor oil and 5 ml/1 tsp camphor oil, shake well to mix. Use to massage the body after a bath.

Skin moisturiser: warm 22 ml/1½ tbsp almond oil and 15 ml/1 tbsp lanolin in a dish over hot water. Add the contents of a vitamin E capsule and 10 ml/2 tsp cold water. Smooth this preparation over the face and neck.

Natural moisturiser for men: combine 10 ml/2 tsp beeswax, 10 ml/2 tsp lanolin, 30 ml/2 tbsp olive oil, 90 ml/6 tbsp infusion of thyme, 12 drops essential oil of cedarwood.

For blackheads: heat 60 ml/4 tbsp honey and add 5 ml/1 tsp wheat-germ, pat over the face and leave on for 10 minutes, wash off with warm water.

For blemishes: blend 15 ml/1 tbsp oatmeal with enough milk to make a paste. Add a whole egg and mix well. Leave on face for 10-15 minutes and rinse first with warm water, then cool.

For cleansing: apply milk of magnesia with cotton wool; leave for 10 minutes, remove and moisturise.

Beauty Products Language

Anti-ageing: these products are formulated to leave the skin feeling and looking softer and smoother but skin aging is biologically irreversible and no externally applied product can change that.

Biodegradable: may appear on shampoo bottles. It only refers to the contents, not the container. It means that 80 per cent of the shampoo will have broken down within 28 days. All shampoos are broken down in time by the elements.

Cruelty-free: animal-friendly or a white rabbit symbol are other labels. This means that the ingredients or the finished product have not been tested on animals in the past five years.

May mean that no animal-derived ingredients have been used.

Dermatologically tested: the product has been tested on human volunteers by using patch tests under strict clinical supervision. Although it was probably tested for tolerance it does not guarantee that it will be suitable for sensitive skin.

Eosin free: may appear on a lipstick case. Eosin is a frequently allergenic colour pigment.

Fragrance free: should be fragrance free, but most of these products contain 0.5per cent perfume.

Green: a very vague term implying the product is biodegradable, not tested on animals and/or environmentally friendly.

Hydrating: generally found on moisturising products. As the term suggests, they help to retain water in the skin.

Hypo-allergenic: the product has been screened for likely irritants and should not contain any well-known allergens.

Jojoba: a natural oil extracted from the jojoba plant, which is used as an alternative to whale oil in skin products for moisturising and lubricating.

Keratin-enriched: hair and nails are made from the protein keratin. Products containing this protein help to strengthen or condition nails or hair.

Liposomes: minute globules which break up in the outer skin layer and help increase the bonding between skin cells. They can be both a component and carrier of ingredients. This term is often found on the label of moisturisers, but their efficacy has been questioned by some dermatologists.

Micronised: on face powder. Means the pigment particles have been very finely ground to give a more even distribution.

Neutralisers: also called free radical scavengers. We have naturally occurring molecules on our skin called free radicals which can be damaging if exposed to the sun or pollutants.

Products containing free radical scavengers, such as vitamin E, vitamin C and selenium neutralise these molecules and thus slow down the ageing process.

Non-acnegenic: claims not to cause aggravation to acne sufferers.

Non-comedogenic: claims to be free of ingredients that block pores and thus cause spots.

Not tested on animals: this particular product or its ingredients have not been tested on animals by their supplier. This term does not guarantee that the ingredients were not tested on animals at some earlier stage of production.

Ozone-friendly: these spray cans should not contain products which contribute to the thinning of the ozone layer.

pH-balanced: in theory, it is beneficial to use skin-care products with a slightly acidic pH, like the skin, to avoid irritation or dryness.

However the skin's natural buffering properties soon revert it to its normal pH-balance, 4.5-5.5, despite the quality of the product used.

Quick-dry formula: a solvent such as alcohol, which evaporates quickly, has been used in the formula to speed up drying time. This may cause allergic reactions in sensitive skin, or have a drying effect on normal skin.

Restructurant: found on hair-care products, claiming to contain ingredients which penetrate the hair and help repair damage.

Most experts agree this is only a temporary cosmetic effect, since hair is composed of dead cells which cannot be revitalised.

Split end repair: the product temporarily binds the split ends of hair back together, thus making it look better. However the only cure is to have the hair trimmed regularly.

Toners: other terminology includes astringents, fresheners and clarifying lotions. These products can be used to clean the last traces of oil from the skin. They do not close or open pores. Sometimes they cause a slight skin irritation which makes the skin feel tighter.

UV filters: used in sun protection products. They absorb or reflect sunlight and displace it as heat thus giving some protection from ultra-violet exposure. The sun protection factor should be indicated by the SPF number on the label.

Many dermatologists believe that premature skin ageing is caused by the sun, since the ultraviolet rays break down the elastic tissues of the skin.

Sunlight may also encourage the production of free radicals. The higher the SPF number the better the protection and the longer you can stay in the sun.

Vitamin-enriched: the value of these products is debatable since it is unknown to what extent vitamins can be absorbed by the skin.

Water-friendly: mainly on hair-care products, this means that the ingredients are not detergent based, but will disperse in water without trace of harmful toxins or resins.

Zinc pyrithione: on anti-dandruff shampoos. This ingredient should alleviate the symptoms of a flaky infected scalp.

Use products containing zinc pyrithione sparingly as it is quite strong and can leave the hair looking very dull and lifeless.

DID YOU KNOW?
You can help prevent wrinkles around your mouth with daily facial exercises. Pull exaggerated O and E shapes with your mouth for 30 seconds.

Purse lips to right, centre and left of your face. Hold each movement for 5 seconds. Repeat three times.

Stick out your tongue as far as you can, keeping you eyes wide. You will feel all the muscles working. Repeat 10 times.

KEEPING HABITS IN CONTROL

Social Drinking

Although an irregular party binge of alcohol will not do any lasting damage, it can make you feel very ill the following day. Here is some advice on how to avoid this situation at that next party.

The amount of time it takes for a person to become intoxicated is relative to their body weight. It is very important to have a good meal beforehand. High-fibre foods such as pasta or wholemeal bread will help absorption.

Drink clear drinks such as white wine or white spirits as 'red' drinks tend to give hangovers.

Never mix alcoholic drinks made from grape with those made from grain. Alternate mineral water or fruit juice with your alcoholic drinks.

Do not keep topping up your drink as you will lose track of how many drinks you have taken.

Mind your glass so that no-one can liven it up without you noticing. If you don't want to drink but people are harassing you, then make the excuse that you are driving or on antibiotics.

Drink a few glasses of water before you go to bed as dehydration is the greatest cause of hangovers. If however you do waken up with a hangover and the two main symptoms of headache and thirst, then the only cure is time and rest. It takes the liver one hour to filter one unit (see below), but it will take another few hours to recover.

Do not be tempted to have another drink, the 'hair of the dog' cure. It will only raise your blood alcohol and is a very dangerous habit which can lead to dependency.

Drink plenty of water, orange juice or sugary drinks. Eat honey. Avoid spicy or acidic foods. When you feel able, it does help to eat a nourishing meal. In particular, alcohol absorbs vitamin B so replenish this with nuts and fruit.

Alkali products may calm your queasy stomach and paracetamol will help the headache but the only cure is patience and time.

DID YOU KNOW?
One unit of alcohol is a glass of wine, ½ pint regular beer or stout, or a single shot of spirits. Men can safely have up to 21 alcohol units spread over a week, while women should only have 14 units.

Stop Smoking

The only way you will give up cigarettes is by convincing yourself that you want to stop smoking. To help this process:

Read the statistics of cancer in the country and do not become oblivious to the health warnings which appear on cigarette packets.

Notice the smell of your clothes after a night out in a smoky atmosphere.

Count how much money you spend on cigarettes.

Realise that the horrible taste in your mouth in the morning is caused by cigarettes and that your breath smells like a used ashtray.

Notice when you have a cold that your symptoms are worse than non-smokers' symptoms. You have a bad cough with revolting sputum.

Remember that if your lung has a slight cut, scratch or raw area on it, each time you inhale smoke it exacerbates that damage.

Try to make the decision to give up cigarettes at a

time when your social calender is quiet and not close to the holiday season. Avoid New Year or Lent; many people try to give up at these times and the failure rate is high. Do not broadcast that you are stopping smoking.

Try 'quit smoking aids' such as nicotine patches but don't replace one dependence with another. Never smoke when using these aids. There are some very good herbal tablet courses that stop the longing for nicotine which is prevalent in the first week.

Your local Health Education Authority will have leaflets giving advice on how to give up cigarettes. You are likely to put on some weight because of your increased appetite and lowered metabolism, so be aware of this tendency and try not to overeat.

If you always had a cigarette with a cup of coffee or tea then substitute this with fruit juice, herbal tea or even eat a piece of fruit. When you do have a cuppa, then read a paper or do the crossword to stop you thinking about the cigarettes.

Start a new routine by doing some new exercise or join an aerobic class. If you are over 30 and have smoked for a long time then consult your doctor about what exercise would be most suitable for you. Learn to relax or meditate for at least 20 minutes each day to avoid stress.

Get busy – start a new hobby, do any jobs that you have left aside for a long time, spring clean or redecorate the house, look outside and see if there is weeding or general work to occupy you.

Try out some new recipes; your smoke-free taste buds will appreciate the new flavours. Avoid nibbling or, if you do, have a bowl of raw fruit or vegetables readily on hand.

Open a new savings account and each week deposit the money you saved by not smoking. Decide how you are going to spend your savings – either buy new clothing for yourself at the end of each month or plan on purchasing a new labour saving appliance. Pick up travel brochures and plan the holiday you've always longed for and make that your aim.

During the first couple of weeks, some people find it relieves the stress to tell their partner or a friend about the agonies they are having without the cigarettes. It is not easy to give up cigarettes and always remember that you are only one cigarette away from being a smoker.

Don't fool yourself; if you take 'just one' cigarette you are back to square one, so find the courage to stay off completely. Remember: if you substitute cigars or pipe smoking for cigarettes, these are just as habit-forming, as dangerous and as anti-social.

There *is* life without cigarettes and when you realise this you are well on the way to freeing yourself from the habit and being a non-smoker.

You will notice an improvement in your general health and fitness and your skin. Smoking can give you wrinkles. The nicotine constricts the flow of blood to the skin, slowing down cell renewal and making wrinkles appear more quickly. It is also suspected to increase free radical production.

Nicotine is also a diuretic drug and dries out the skin, making any existing facial lines more obvious. Tiny lines form around the mouth as a result of sucking cigarettes. The skin ageing process is also accelerated because cigarette smoking encourages the production of free radicals.

Sleep Tight

There are many theories on how many hours sleep we need. Lying awake worrying that we are not having enough sleep only intensifies the problem. The best time to go to bed is when you are tired and ready to go to sleep. A few hours before bedtime get some fresh air or go for a short walk. If you feel a little bit cold going to bed, you may find that the warmth of a heated bed will make you relaxed and sleepy.

If soft music helps you relax, many radio alarms can switch off automatically after an hour, so you have no worry about the radio being on all night.

About an hour before you go to bed start winding down. Read a book, write a letter or listen to music rather than watch a gripping TV programme. A warm bath is always relaxing; try adding a few drops of lavender or marjoram oil.

Only use your bedroom for sleeping; do not work, read or watch television. If you are not asleep after half an hour, get up and leave the room.

In bed try consciously relaxing each part of your body in turn, slowly working up from your toes.

To avoid becoming preoccupied with your inability to sleep, try counting backwards from 100, or go through the alphabet and find a different thing you like for each letter. Think of how you would spend a windfall of a few thousand pounds.

Some people find that it helps to have a regular routine of going to bed and getting up at set times.

Do not eat a heavy meal before going to bed. A warm milky drink will make you feel sleepy but soft drinks, coffee or alcohol should not be taken late at night as they increase mental activity. Have a notepad and pencil by your bed to note down any preoccupations or reminders.

Get up earlier in the morning and you will find that you are tired at bedtime. Keep the bedroom pleasantly warm but not stuffy. Use heavy curtains on the windows and you will not be awakened by the dawn light.

For chronic insomniacs, research has developed a method that is quite successful. You must have a week free to allow you to sleep during the day.

The idea is to alter the body's natural sleep rhythm from its later sleep pattern to an earlier one thus bringing it back to normal. This rhythm can be more easily altered by extending the waking day so you go to bed later each day and after six days bedtime is back to normal.

For example: you are not going to sleep normally until 4 or 5 am. The first night stay awake until 7.30 am. The second night stay awake until 11 am and continue to extend your bedtime to 2 pm, 5 pm, 8 pm, ending up going to bed at 11 pm on the sixth day. Keep going to bed at 11 pm and your sleep pattern should settle at this time.

Stress Control

Excessive stress and tension can affect your health so keep them under control. Avoid working more than 10 hours a day. Take at least one day off work every week to spend at leisure. Avoid rushing; get up 15-20 minutes earlier and enjoy the morning. If your work schedule for the day is an extra-long list of duties, don't panic. Select what is urgent and deal with it first. The rest can be done if you have time or maybe even kept for another day.

Take some time for yourself every day. Know how you are going to spend this break. Perhaps there's a book you have been wanting to read or some craft or hobby you want to try. Plan and enjoy every minute of your break.

Concentrate on the present. Stop dwelling on the past or worrying about the future. Learn to say 'no'. Too many favours or too much voluntary work can leave you without any free time for yourself.

Don't compete with your friends, neighbours or workmates. Be your own person and live your life according to your own principles.

Be realistic and avoid setting unattainable goals; this will only cause frustration. Probably the most important factor is how you feel about yourself.

Exercise at least three times a week. Physical activities – sports, walking, jogging, aerobics or gardening– are excellent ways to relieve tension.

When you feel under pressure and tense, count slowly to 20. Watch out for jaw, neck and shoulder tension and learn consciously to relax these areas.

'Smile and the whole world smiles with you.' Be pleasant to people around you. Kind words of appreciation to others make you feel good. Have fun and laughter – a good sense of humour is good medicine for stress. There's pleasure in giving as well as receiving, so enjoy doing kind deeds.

Stop being obstinate and learn to give in. There is generally a way around most things. Learn to express your feelings and emotions openly, without unnecessary aggression.

Often problems are the cause of stress. There's a saying that 'a problem shared is a problem halved' and this is very true. Find someone you can trust: a religious minister, a professional helper, a relative or a friend. Talk over your problem with them and you may find that a different approach could solve your worries.

Try not to be a perfectionist in everything – no-one is perfect. Take a look at yourself and think of all your good points. When you're dealing with other people look out for their good points. Avoid always being critical and negative.

Drink plenty of water – at least eight glasses a day. Eat a healthy diet (high fibre, low fat) with regular mealtimes. Reduce your caffeine and sugar intake. Alcohol and cigarettes do not relieve stress – they sometimes exacerbate it.

Drugs used to control stress can become addictive very quickly. They may relieve some of the obvious symptoms but do nothing to change your way of life or your behaviour. Learn relaxation techniques and practice them daily. Some people find meditation helpful. Try to have at least one holiday away from your work and home environment every year; do not turn self-catering holidays into work.

> **DID YOU KNOW?**
> An American insurance company found that if a wife simply kisses her husband goodbye each morning she increases his life expectancy.

THE MEDICINE CHEST

First-Aid Kits

Every home should have a first-aid box stocked with emergency first-aid materials. It should be kept where it is easily available. Other materials and preparations should be kept in a locked medicine cabinet with the key close to hand. The labelled box should contain the following items:

Assorted adhesive plasters
Gauze
Roll of adhesive plaster
Cotton wool
A selection of bandages
Scissors
Antiseptic ointment
Safety pins
Antiseptic solution
Burn wipes/spray

The locked medicine cupboard should have:

Calamine lotion
Soluble aspirin
Soothing eye lotion
Antacid medicine
Paracetemol tablets/liquid
Cough linctus
Kaolin mixture
Vapour rub
Antiseptic throat lozenges
Laxatives
Travel sickness tablets
Deep heat rub

In case of emergency, have the details of the local doctor and hospital handy by the telephone and be aware of any limitations regarding the hours and services of your local casualty unit.

Note information on family health: past illnesses and subsequent treatment, dates of operations or hospital treatments, allergies and long-term use of medication, and any immunisations.

Relieve a headache with a massage: press firmly with both index and middle fingers into the base of the head where the skull joins the spine. Hold for seven seconds and repeat three times. Then rub both temples in small circular motions, first in one direction then in the other, with the same fingers.

To relieve muscular tension, press moist compresses to the forehead and hot compresses to the neck and shoulders.

Alternative First Aid

Natural doesn't always mean safe. Herbs can be potent so they should be used with great care. Do not exceed the recommended dose for any herbal preparation. If you are pregnant do not take any herbal preparation without consulting your doctor.

Do not mix herbal medications with conventional ones without consulting your general practitioner.

Never take home remedies for more than two weeks without seeking medical attention.

To make a **poultice**: mash or grate the ingredients, mix them with enough hot water to make a thick paste. Smear this over a sterile dressing pad and place a piece of clean gauze over it.

Apply it as hot as bearable to the affected area and leave it in place until it is cool.

Baking soda: when stung by an insect, first remove any remaining sting with a pair of tweezers.

Avoid squeezing the poison sac as this pushes the remaining poison into the skin.

Bee and ant stings: apply a solution of baking soda and water, while for wasp stings use vinegar. Dry the area and cover with a cold compress.

If stung in the mouth, suck an ice cube or rinse the mouth with a solution of cold water and baking soda. Repeat as required.

Watch out for swelling, which can cause breathing difficulties. A severe allergic reaction to a sting may result in a state of shock, requiring urgent medical help. To remember which sting cure to use: 'B is for Baking Soda'; 'V in vinegar' and 'W in wasp' are similar in shape.

For cystitis: at the first signs of an attack, drink a glass of water with 5ml/1tsp added baking soda, every hour for three hours.

Barley water: for diarrhoea, try Mrs Beeton's recipe : 50 g/2 oz pearl barley, 2/3 lumps sugar, thinly pared rind of half a lemon and 600 ml/1 pint boiling water. Cover barley with cold water, boil for 2 minutes and strain. Place the barley, sugar and lemon rind in a jug, pour in 600 ml/1 pint boiling water and cover. Strain when cold and use to replenish lost fluid and energy or mix with ready-made rehydration medication sachets to make them more palatable.

Camomile flower tea: use instead of painkillers for a headache or to calm the nerves.

Carrot: for sties, grate a carrot finely and put into a piece of muslin or a fine cotton handkerchief. Dab on the sty frequently until it comes to a head.

Cayenne pepper: use on cuts or minor wounds. It will sting but promotes rapid healing.

Cider vinegar: for a sore throat, add 5 ml/1 tsp cider vinegar to a glass of water and gargle. Alternatively gargle with a glass of water containing 5 ml/1 tsp each salt and baking soda or chew a piece of raw onion.

Garlic: peel a clove of garlic and cut off a slice. Place the cut end on a mouth ulcer and squeeze the juice onto it. For corns, crush a garlic clove and put onto the corn. Cover with a plaster or bandage. Renew daily. To remove garlic from the breath, chew a clove or some fresh parsley.

Herbal tea: elderflower, lemon, peppermint or balm teas all help to relax the body.

Honey: a natural healer for cuts and burns. Very good for sore or chapped lips.

Ice-pack: apply to sprains for fast relief. Use cubes or crushed ice in a strong plastic bag or a bag of frozen vegetables; wrap in a towel or cloth. Only use the ice-pack for 20 minutes at a time. Never use on blisters or wounds, if the patient has circulatory problems or is hypersensitive to cold.

Lemon juice: for constipation, before breakfast every day, drink a glass of warm water with a little lemon juice added. For hayfever or that stuffed-up feeling, mix a few drops lemon with a few drops hot water and inhale with each nostril.

Lettuce: to reduce swelling and soreness from a bruise, tape washed lettuce leaves over the affected area. Apply fresh leaves every few hours.

For a sprained ankle or wrist, use a hot lettuce poultice to stop swelling.

Onion: to cure chilblains, rub twice daily with a slice of onion dipped in salt.

Oil of cloves or garlic: to relieve toothache, soak a piece of cotton wool and pack next to the painful tooth while awaiting urgent dental attention.

Parsley: chew parsley to remove the smell of garlic from the breath or to relieve flatulence.

Salt water: this is one of the most effective solutions for cleansing and will help to heal minor wounds and cuts. Use a solution of 5 ml/1 tsp salt in 250 ml/8 fl oz hot water.

This solution can also be used to ease the mouth after a tooth extraction. Cool the liquid, roll it around the mouth, then spit it out. A salt water gargle will ease a sore throat.

Tincture of cayenne: rub on painful gums.

Thyme and tea tree oil: will clean a wound and stop infection but will also sting.

Water: speedy immersion in water for at least two minutes is essential for minor burns. Then treat with a mixture of one part lemon juice and three parts water. Apply with cotton wool.

Other remedies for minor burns are milk of magnesia or a paste of bicarbonate of soda and water. It is essential to get medical attention for severe burns as soon as possible.

Home-Grown Medicine

Arthritis: drink parsley tea, an infusion made with 250 ml/8 fl oz boiling water and 5 ml/1 tsp chopped parsley. Let it infuse until cool, strain and sip throughout the day.

Baby colic: crush 5 ml/1 tsp caraway, dill or fennel seeds, soak 250 ml/8 fl oz boiling water for half an hour; strain and use when necessary.

Boils: Never squeeze or burst a boil. To get rid of one, you must draw it to a head using a hot poultice. Make one from either a slice of bread and hot water or an onion peeled and baked until soft. Place the poultice on the boil and leave until cool. When the boil bursts, clean away the pus with plenty of clean swabs.

Bruises: eat fresh pineapple or drink pineapple juice to help bruises heal. Vinegar, witch hazel and ice are all useful for applying to bruises.

Chapped lips: mix 75 ml/5 tbsp almond oil with 15 ml/1 tbsp melted beeswax. Rub on as required.

Cold sores: mix 5 ml/1 tsp vodka with 2 drops each of tea tree, bergamot and eucalyptus oils. Dab on the sore regularly as required during the day to stop a blister forming.

Cold prevention: squeeze juice of half a lemon into 300 ml/½ pint hot water, add 5 ml/1 tsp honey to sweeten and 1 pinch cinnamon.

Simmer a large onion in milk until very soft, eat the onion and drink the milk. Alternatively, slice an onion onto a plate, sprinkle with sugar, leave for an hour until the juice is extracted. Sip the juice.

Put 2.25 litres/4 pints hot water into a basin and add 6 ml/1 heaped tsp dried mustard. Soak feet in this for 10 minutes before going to bed.

Steep 6 ml/1 heaped tsp elderflowers in 250 ml/ 8 fl oz boiling water for 20 minutes. Strain, add honey to taste and drink hot at bedtime.

Common cold: using a heat resistant glass, add one or two peeled and crushed cloves of garlic, half the grated rind and all the juice of one lemon, a pinch of cayenne pepper, 2.5 ml/½ tsp ground powdered ginger and 15 ml/1 tbsp honey. Stir well to mix and add 250 ml/8 fl oz nearly boiling water.

Allow to cool and then drink the whole lot, including the solids, and go straight to bed.

The basis of this preparation is garlic, which is noted for its power in inhibiting the growth of bacteria such as streptococcus.

The lemon acts on the mucus membrane of the nose and alleviates the symptoms of nasal congestion or constant dripping. The ginger increases the heat in the digestion area, which boosts the blood supply and secretory juices, which aid the expulsion of catarrh into the bowel. The pinch of cayenne pepper is a trigger on the stored Vitamin C in the body. The honey soothes and heals the raw tissue areas.

This combination causes profuse sweating so it is sensible to stay in bed until the sweating stops. The sleep and rest will help to aid recovery.

Congestion of the chest: add some peppermint essence or friar's balsam to a bowl of boiling water. Drape a towel over your head and lean over the bowl, staying at least 22 cm/9 inches above the water. Inhale the steam for 5 minutes to loosen any mucus in the nose or throat and help you breathe more easily. Not suitable for sensitive skin, since the steam can cause broken veins.

An Indian remedy that is successful in clearing catarrh causing a cough or bronchitis: put 5 ml/ 1 tsp turmeric in a saucepan with 250 ml/8 fl oz milk and bring to the boil. Sweeten with sugar or honey to taste. Drink this mixture three times a day. There should be a marked change within the course of three days. Note that turmeric is bright yellow and will stain certain utensils and crockery.

Coughs: add 5 cloves peeled and crushed garlic to 225 ml/8 fl oz honey. Cover and leave to stand for 24 hours. Take 5 ml/1 tsp hourly.

Put into a bottle 110 g/4 oz pure cod liver oil, 110g/4 oz pure honey, 25 g/1 oz glycerine and the strained juice of three lemons. Shake well before pouring and take the mixture three times a day after meals.

Make a garlic syrup by crushing 250 g/9 oz garlic and adding it to 1 litre/1.75 pint jar. Fill with equal amounts water and cider. Cover and leave for a few days, stirring occasionally. Strain, then add 250 ml/8 fl oz honey. Store in the fridge and take 15 ml/1 tbsp three times a day.

Relieve a troublesome night cough by drinking a glass of hot milk containing 5 ml/1 tsp black treacle or molasses and a pinch of nutmeg.

A dry irritating cough: to 200 ml/⅓ pint boiling water add the juice of one lemon, 10 ml/2 tsp honey, 1.25 ml/¼ tsp cinnamon, 1 clove garlic and a sprig of rosemary. Stir well, cover and leave for 15 minutes. Strain and sip slowly. Alternatively, fill a mug two-thirds full with hot milk, melt a knob of butter on top. Drink the mixture without stirring. Add a little nutmeg or cinnamon if required.

Constipation: soak dried prunes overnight in water or orange juice or poach them in apple juice. Eat with a high fibre cereal for breakfast.

Cystitis: pour 250 ml/8 fl oz boiling water over 5 ml/1 tsp powdered marshmallow root. Stir and leave for 20 minutes. Add 5 ml/1 tsp honey and take the mixture three times a day before meals. To ward off cystitis, drink cranberry juice daily.

Diarrhoea: in some cultures the recommended cure is to eat only well-cooked salted rice and to drink the water it was cooked in until the problem clears. For children with diarrhoea give plenty of flat cola or lemonade. To make the mineral flat, pour it into a glass and stir vigorously, or leave the bottle uncorked for several hours.

Eczema: steep 15 g/½ oz camomile flowers in 600 ml/1 pint boiling water for 20 minutes and add to the bath for relief.

Fatigue/exhaustion: sprinkle a few basil leaves into a hot bath or wrap leaves in muslin and hold under the hot tap. It may also help to drink a mug of basil infusion in the morning. Sweeten to taste.

Hayfever: several months before the hayfever season, start taking 15 ml/1 tbsp natural comb honey three times a day.

Headaches: drink an infusion of rosemary to relieve a tension headache, colds or flu.

Hiccups: make a drink with 10 ml/2 tsp crushed dill seeds in a little hot water, infuse for a few minutes, strain and dilute with cold water. Other traditional cures are to swallow 5 ml/1 tsp vinegar, to chew fresh mint leaves or eat 10 ml/2 tsp orange marmalade.

Indigestion and flatulence: use plenty of rosemary, bay leaves, thyme, sage or marjoram when cooking your savoury dishes.

Drinking caraway, fennel seed or camomile tea after meals can also aid digestion. Chew basil leaves or sip 125 ml/4 fl oz milk simmered with 5 ml/1tsp honey and some nutmeg. Sip an infusion of 5 ml/1 tsp finely grated root ginger in 250 ml/ 8 fl oz hot water.

Alternatively, to reduce acidity, dissolve 5 ml/1 tsp bicarbonate of soda in a glass of water. Do not take this too often as over a period of time the stomach will produce more acid to compensate.

Insomnia: eat a boiled onion or drink hop, catnip or camomile tea at bedtime.

Menopause: take an infusion of basil to help alleviate problems of irritability and forgetfulness.

Mouth ulcer: apply glycerine every two hours to the ulcer. After meals rinse the mouth with a solution of warm water and baking soda. Yogurt can also be used as a treatment. At bedtime take 15 ml/1 tbsp unsweetened natural yogurt and hold it in the mouth for as long as possible, especially over the affected area. Do not rinse.

Mouthwash or gargle: pour 600 ml/1 pint boiling water over 6 ml/1 heaped tsp dried sage, cover and leave for 10 minutes. Strain and use hot.

Nappy rash: soak 5 ml/1 tsp dried elderflowers or 10 ml/2 tsp fresh flowers in 600 ml/1 pint boiling water. Cover and leave for 20 minutes. When cool apply to the affected area with sterile gauze.

Nausea and travel sickness: infuse 2.5 ml/½ tsp
grated ginger in 250 ml/8 fl oz boiling water for a
few minutes. Strain and drink.

Period pains: use an infusion of dried marigold
flower heads to help relieve period pains.
A tincture of marigold is useful in regulating the
menstrual cycle.

Stomach upset: simmer 5 ml/1 tsp cinnamon and
honey in water for 20 minutes, cool and sip slowly.
For an acid stomach make meadowsweet tea and
sip after meals.

Tiredness and fatigue: pour 250 ml/8 fl oz boiling
water over 5 ml/1 tsp rosemary leaves, infuse for
half an hour and strain. Drink half a cup, warm,
first thing in the morning and at bedtime. As a
general tonic, infuse a handful of dandelion leaves
in 600 ml/1 pint boiling water for 10 minutes.
Strain and drink three cups daily.

Revitalising rosehip tonic: cover 1.75 kg/4 lb
rosehips with water and bring to the boil. Simmer
until soft. Put the pulp into a muslin bag and
squeeze out the juice. Return to pan and repeat.

Add all the juice to a clean muslin bag, and let it
drip into a basin, then add 900 g/2 lb sugar, stir and
boil for five minutes. Bottle and seal immediately.
Take 5 ml/1 tsp daily as a tonic during the winter.

Sinus trouble: inhale a few drops of peppermint or
eucalyptus oil from a tissue. If congestion is severe,
use the fingertips to press along the cheekbones

from the nose to the temple after inhaling the oil. Alternatively, drink an infusion of 5 ml/1 tsp marjoram in 250 ml/8 fl oz boiling water two or three times a day. If symptoms remain after 24 hours, consult your doctor.

Thorns: most thorns will ease out with a hot bath and squeezing. If this fails, sterilise a needle and gently open the skin over the thorn, squeeze and remove the thorn with tweezers. Bathe the area with witch hazel.

Failing this, mix castor oil, which should be as hot as the skin can bear, with flour and apply. Cover with a bandage for 12 hours. The thorn should come out easily.

Thrush: often occurs after a course of antibiotics. If in the mouth eat plain yogurt. In the vaginal area, cleanse with olive oil, not water. Insert natural yogurt into the vagina with fingertips or on a tampon. Be sure to remove the tampon.

An infusion of camomile used as a douche twice daily will help to soothe the area. Boil garlic cloves and use the cooled water on a compress.

Tongue burn: if you burn your tongue with hot coffee or tea, soothe it by sprinkling a little sugar onto the tip.

Tooth extraction: after having a tooth removed, use an infusion of lady's mantle or camomile flowers to rinse out the mouth and as a gargle.

Travel sickness: chew a small piece of ginger or suck ginger-flavoured sweets.

Varicose veins: apply a compress of marigold flower decoction to the affected area and very gently massage upwards.

Warts: pour 150 ml/¼ pint boiling water over 50 g/2 oz ivy leaves. Cool and strain. Dampen a piece of cotton wool with the ivy water, apply to the wart and cover with a plaster twice daily.

Another remedy is to rub the wart daily with lemon juice. Both treatments should gradually soften the wart and it will fall off.

You and Your Doctor

When you move to an new area it is advisable to register with a local doctor as soon as possible. Do not wait until an emergency arises.

Ask your previous doctor for a short medical record of your family for the new practitioner.

Ask neighbours or residents in the area about the reputations of local doctors. Go to the surgery and meet the reception staff and, if possible, the doctor.

It may take a few visits before you become relaxed and comfortable with a new practice.

Take note of the surgery hours, information on appointments and special clinics available such as ante-natal or injection times for children.

Enquire on the procedure when the doctor is off duty, and get any necessary phone numbers. Find out if essential home visits are available.

When visiting the doctor, make a list of all the matters you wish to discuss. With any specific complaint be clear when the symptoms started, where and how bad they are and what, if anything, makes them worse.

Give precise details; do not exaggerate or minimise details – let the doctor decide their importance. Be prepared to undress for examination quickly.

If you do not understand the doctor's terminology, ask for an explanation in layman's terms.

Always tell the doctor about any consultations you have had with other medical practitioners since your last visit.

Prescribed Drugs

Make sure the doctor knows if you are allergic to any treatment and let him or her know about any alternative medicine you might use.

When you are prescribed drugs it is important that you ask the doctor to explain why he prescribed the drug and what it is supposed to do.

Perhaps there is some literature on the drug he could give you. Find out the generic or full name of the drug as well as the brand name.

Know how to take the medication:
Should it be taken before or with meals, by itself or
with a drink of water, milk or tea?

Should it be sucked, chewed or swallowed whole,
and how often should it be taken?

Should the times be spaced out over 24 hours or
just waking hours?

If you forget a dose, should you take a double dose
next time?

How long do you continue with the medication
and will you need a repeat prescription?

What are the potential side-effects and what
should you do if you experience any of these?

Is it advisable to take other drugs such as
painkillers at the same time?

If there is an increase or decrease in symptoms
should you change the prescribed dose accordingly?

Should you have a further check-up on finishing
the course even though you feel well again?

Check that the chemist has written all the relative
information on the medication label.

It is very important to complete the full course of
any prescribed medicine. This is particularly true
of antibiotics.

HEALTHIER EATING

Food Jargon

Since the introduction of high technology in food production and mass distribution, most foodstuffs now contain some of these additives:

Colourings (E100-E180) rarely add to the nutritional value of foods but are merely cosmetic and are often used to disguise the poor quality of ingredients in processed foods. Generally synthetic colours are used because they are cheaper and more stable than the natural kind.

Preservatives (E200-E299) inhibit the growth of micro-organisms such as bacteria, yeasts and moulds. They also deactivate enzymes which lead to the deterioration of food.

Natural preservatives are sugar, salt, vinegar, alcohol and wood smoke.

Synthetic preservatives include potassium nitrate and sodium nitrate, used in cured and cooked meats to prevent botulism and to give an attractive pink colour to meat products.

Nisin is an antibiotic used in cheese. Phenyls prevent fungal growth on the surface of citrus fruit but may be absorbed as far as the pulp. Sulphur dioxide is used to preserve fruit juices, cider, beer and wine.

All these synthetic additives are widely used despite scientific concerns about their safety.

Antioxidants (E300-E321) prevent oxidation (chemical deterioration when exposed to the oxygen in the air) of certain foods, especially oily or fat products. Rancid food does not only taste and smell bad; it can also be unsafe to eat.

Natural antioxidants are ascorbic acid (vitamin C), E300, and tocopherols (vitamin E), E306.

Two common synthetic antioxidants are butylated hydroxyanisole (BHA), E320, and butylated hydroxytoluene (BHT), E321.

These two synthetic additives are subject to intensive safety research and are often proclaimed as being the cause of hives and hyperactivity in children. Since they are used as processing aids, they may not always be declared on the label.

Emulsifiers and stabilisers (E322-495) make up the largest group of additives. Emulsifiers are used to bind together two substances such as oil and water which normally repel each other.

They help to incorporate the air into the liquid when processing ice-cream, while in puddings and milk shakes they are used as a thickening agent, making the finished product bulkier.

Stabilisers prevent the mixtures from separating as well as being a thickening agent.

Many of these additives are from natural substances and are accepted as perfectly safe. However some synthesised emulsifiers and stabilisers can be suspect and often their only function is to increase the weight or volume of the finished product.

Sometimes manufacturers add nutrients to foods to replace those lost during processing. These include many of the vitamins and calcium.

Acids, bases and others (500-529) are used as raising agents, preservatives or to give a tart flavour to food. Bases increase alkalinity.

Anti-caking agents and others (530-578) are chemicals added to granular or powdered foods to prevent them sticking together through the absorption of moisture.

They can also stop processed foods from adhering to the machinery during processing. These agents are generally not declared on the label.

Flavour enhancers, sweeteners (620-637) have little or no flavour in themselves but enhance the flavour of other foods and improve its edibility by stimulating the taste buds.

Often refined sugar used in processing is labelled as a food. However it has no nutritional value since as a result of severe refining it becomes a chemical substance.

It would be difficult to estimate how much 'hidden' processed sugar is used in products.

Glazing agents (900-907) are waxes and oils used to put a shine on foods such as dried fruit or sweets. They will not be mentioned on the label if they are used on the raw ingredients in another product, for example the dried fruit in a cereal.

Bleaching agents and improvers (920-927) are used to whiten and sterilise flour and bread products. These increase the shelf life but remove the nutrients, lowering the nutritional value. They may not appear on the label.

Unnumbered additives: there are a whole range of these used in the production of foodstuffs but not declared on the label.

Not all of these have been tested and the safety of some of them has been questioned by some scientists. Since the consumer is not given any information on these additives it is impossible to know when or where they are used.

When there is an E before the number this shows that the additive has been approved by the European Union (EU). A number on its own means that the additive is permitted in some European countries but is not yet approved by the EU. Many of these are being considered for approval but others may eventually be banned.

The label on many products gives a limited amount of information if you can decipher the codes. Several types of food do not have an ingredients label, however. These include most dairy products, fresh fruit and vegetables, some confectionery and many alcoholic drinks. Sometimes the description of the product will give you an idea of the contents: 'fruit flavour' means artificial flavour, 'fruit flavoured' means that a small amount of fruit was used, whereas a 'fruit product' contains a substantial amount of fruit.

Often you will see 'Free from artificial flavourings, colourings and preservatives' written on a label. This statement may be misleading.

For example, on checking the small print on the label you may see that the product contains a flavour enhancer such as 621 – monosodium gluta-mate (MSG). This is used as a substitute for more expensive ingredients; it enhances the flavours of synthesised foods.

MSG is prohibited in foods intended for young children but is frequently found in processed foods such as fish fingers, beef burgers, sausages, packet soups, crisps and other convenience foods.

Many flavourings are chemically synthesised but are called 'nature identical' because they have the same chemical structure as the natural flavour.

Some 'natural' colourings can be unhealthy, for example, caramel (E150). You may associate this with burnt sugar; however, it is mostly made with ammonia and/or sulphite yet still labelled 'natural'.

Manufacturers of medicines do not have to declare colourings or additives. Children's medicines often contain colouring and a high sugar content.

Unless you have a very restricted diet and shop daily then additives will play a part in your daily nourishment. It is worthwhile learning about the additives you are consuming and know what to look for on the labels of products.

Many fresh food products are additive-free but you will find that most of them have been grown on land fertilised with man-made fertilizers or sprayed with chemicals to prolong their life or simply to improve their appearance. Organic food, if properly produced, should be grown on land that has been free from chemical fertilizers and sprays for a period of at least two years.

On labels, ingredients are listed in descending order of weight. If sugar is the first ingredient then the product contains more sugar than anything else. However, sometimes sugar is given names such as fructose, corn syrup, glucose syrup, and although it may be the principal ingredient it will be split up under the various different names.

Water only has to be listed if it is more than 5 per cent of the total weight. However many meat products are treated with polyphosphates to absorb the water content.

Processed foods account for 70-80 per cent of our salt intake. Foods high in salt are cheese, bacon, ham, tinned and packet soups, crisps, salted peanuts, smoked meats and fish, baking powder, tinned fish, foods that contain monosodium glutamate (MSG) or saccharin, soda water and yeast extracts.

A high intake of salt in the diet can substantially raise blood pressure and the risk of heart attack.

Healthy Cuisine

When shopping for food: only shop for food where the staff and premises are hygienic. Avoid counters that have raw and cooked foods displayed together. Disposable gloves should be worn by assistants when handling any food. Do not buy food from an assistant who is handling both money and food.

Cheese should not be dry looking. Buy only small quantities and avoid buying cheese wrapped in plastic-film packets. Cheese should never be stored directly next to meat.

Stone fruits such as peaches or plums should be firm and not bruised. They are best eaten the day of purchase but can be kept for a day if they are bought a little under-ripe.

Windfall apples or pears usually have bruises and will rot when stored. However, they can be cooked and the purée frozen.

Vegetables should also be fresh when purchased to ensure a high vitamin content as well as the best taste. In addition to looking for plumpness and brightness, check that the vegetables smell fresh.

Freshness is essential when purchasing fish – the flesh should be firm, the eyes clear, shiny and full, the gills bright red and it should smell clean. Avoid fish that looks pallid or has skin with a blue or green tinge. Bright silvery trout are a better buy than ones with a black or reddish appearance. Fresh shellfish should look crisp and dry. Broken mussels, scallops, oysters or those that remain open when tapped should be discarded.

Remember when you purchase meat, the colour is not a guarantee of the quality – it is only an indication. Sometimes meat on display looks redder and juicier than it actually is, as a result of the warm lighting. As a general rule, beef should be plum red, pork a pale pink, and lamb should be pink tinged with red. The fat should be creamy to white depending on the meat. Poultry and game should look firm and shiny, with no bruises.

Check the best-before and sell-by date on packet labels. 'Sell-by' dates are printed at the discretion of the manufacturer. 'Eat-by' means eat by that date, subject to correct storage. 'Best before' means eat by the end of the day of the printed date.

Avoid dented or swollen tins, damaged packets or fresh food that has been stored or displayed in direct sunlight.

Check what your food purchases are stored beside. Strong smelling goods can taint those alongside them. In particular, eggs with their porous shells are vulnerable to other smells.

Do not buy frozen food from an over-filled chest freezer. Buy frozen or chilled foods last when shopping and if your journey home takes more than an hour, use a cool bag.

Determined Dieting

Calories act as fuel for the body. If you regularly ingest more calories than your body requires the surplus is stored as extra fat. Thus, you may find it particularly difficult to control your weight if you lead a sedentary lifestyle and take very little exercise .

To stay slim, you have to get the proper balance between the calories you consume and the calories you burn up. The body deals in different ways with calories from different foods. It uses more calories to break down carbohydrates and proteins than when dealing with fats. So a low-fat diet not only means a lower consumption of calories, but that more are burned up during digestion.

For this reason it is sensible to eat main meals earlier in the day so that the calories are burned up by daily activity. Avoid eating late meals as they are more easily turned into body fat. For practical reasons and also to avoid the feeling of hunger, it is best to space the calorie intake evenly during the day, up to early evening.

Choose your slimming diet carefully. Many fad diets are nutritionally inadequate as they do not include enough minerals and vitamins.

Calorie-controlled diets will reduce weight, but to keep slim, more success can be achieved by the adjustment of eating habits. It is easy to start a diet but very difficult to keep it up unless it is taken as normal lifestyle.

Like giving up smoking or alcohol, each person must make up her or his own mind that they want to lose weight, and be very determined to do so. Don't look at a diet régime as a punishment; think positively about the benefits you will gain.

Set realistic goals. You may need to lose 12 kg/2 stones; aim to lose 6 kg/1 stone first, then tackle the rest. Some people might find that small weekly targets are more easily attainable.

Look at your present eating habits. Keep a food diary and take note of everything you eat and drink, time and place of meals, your mood, what you are doing while you eat and if you are alone or in company. Be very honest.

From your diary ascertain your eating pattern. See where you eat unnecessarily and how you can avoid this in future.

Check with your doctor to discuss a suitable form of exercise you will enjoy. Get into the routine of doing a workout three or four times a week.

When you start the new eating regime:
Do not shop when you are hungry. Make a list of the goods you require and stick to it rigidly. Keep all tempting foods out of view when you open the fridge or cupboard.

Gradually remove all sweet goods, high-fat and salty foods from your shopping list. It will take time for your tastebuds to adjust if you are used to eating lots of junk food.

Increase your purchases of wholemeal bread,
potatoes and cereals, pulses and fish, vegetables
and fresh fruit. Include plenty of high fibre foods in
your diet. These include bread, rice, cereals,
vegetables, fruit and nuts. Aim for about 30 g/1 oz
of fibre a day.

Eat slowly and enjoy the food at the dining table
rather than in front of the television so that
attention is paid to the plate of food. An average
meal should take at least 20 minutes to eat so the
brain can register that 'full' feeling.

Avoid foods with a hidden fat content. Cut down
on fatty red meats, substituting fish and poultry.
Rather than frying food, grill, bake or steam it.
Substitute semi-skimmed or skimmed milk for
full-fat milk and use reduced-fat spreads rather
than butter or margarine.

Use herbs and spices imaginatively to make your
diet taste more interesting. Grate or chop fruit and
vegetables to make the quantity look larger and use
smaller plates to make the portions seem bigger.
Never eat leftovers; either use them for another
meal, feed them to the dog or discard them. If
you still feel hungry after a meal, don't be tempted
to eat extra, if you have already used up your
daily calorie allowance. Get into the habit of
saying 'no' politely but firmly when encouraged to
take extra helpings.

Have available low calorie foods such as fruit or
raw vegetables to nibble to combat hunger pangs.
Don't fool yourself – 'diet' foods still contain

calories so limit their use. Read labels with care – some foods considered 'healthy', such as unsweetened fruit juice, can have 50 kcal per 50 ml/2 fl oz. Avoid alcohol, especially with high-calorie mixers – the calories in it have no nutritional value and it may increase your appetite.

Keep a chart of your body measurements - bust, tops of arms, waist, hips and tops of thighs. Every three weeks enter the new measurements. When you have 2.5 cm/1 inch off your waist and hips, reward your results by buying a new outfit. Save for the spending spree by putting aside an amount of money equal to the weight that you have lost.

Don't become obsessed with the scales. Weigh yourself only once a week at the same time of the day. This is still only a guide, as fluid retention can vary and women in particular will retain more water at certain times of their monthly cycle.

Some people find they have more incentive to slim if they join a group for moral support.

DID YOU KNOW?
A calorie is the unit value of the amount of heat energy 'given off' food if it was burnt. A joule is the measurement of the energy expended by the body to function. Since calories and joules are such tiny measurements, the energy content of food, stated on labels, is measured in thousands of units. Thus they are called kilocalories (Kcal) and kilojoules (Kj). One Kcal equals 4.18 Kj.

INDEX